This Book is dedicated to:

Shining a light of Thereupeutic empathy onto
Terres des Hommes world; via Theriault VIP
Concierge <u>15 essentials walk-through</u> guide
so as to get
you to the church
on time Daddi...

Chapter 1: Stop streamin`
Empty Calories life is short

Make time to stream these total Breathwork guides you use to breath in nose and out through the lips through like ebb flow of tide yet all calm beneath the surface like your own personal <u>Ayahausca Mantra visuelle</u>

<u>That easy: View Motion Graphic Monoliths for Breathwork Syn`c here.</u>
<u>Then read on with wild abandom Johnny Boy</u>

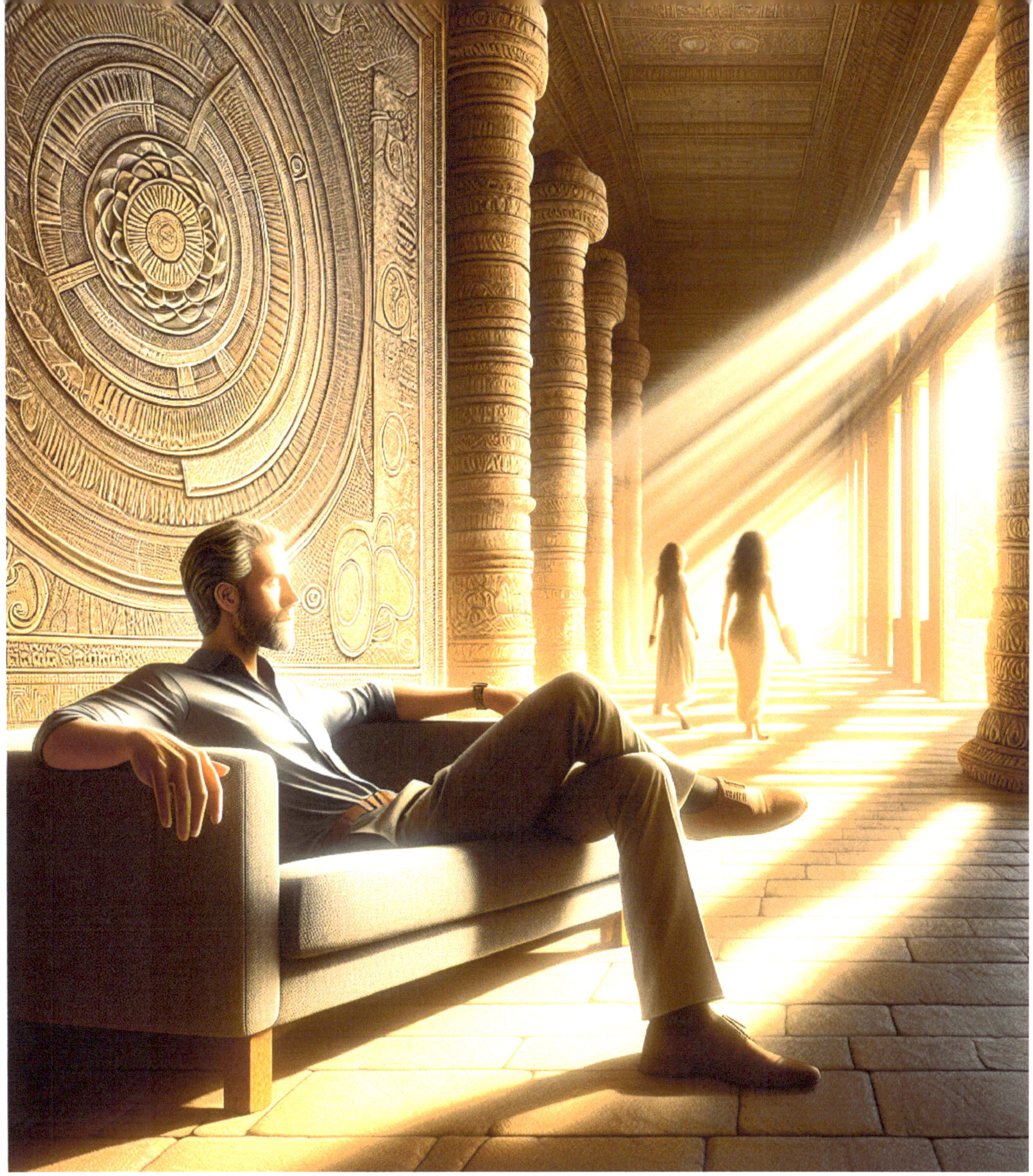

Chapter 2: Fortify the Blood
with the man root tonic

Korean Red Ginseng is a natural and powerful way to promote your overall well-being. Thanks to its ginsenosides and saponins, it offers multiple health benefits, including reducing inflammation, improving brain function, fighting fatigue, boosting immunity, protecting against cancer, and improving erectile dysfunction. It's important to note that American and Asian ginseng differ in their concentration of active compounds and effects on the body. While American ginseng works as a relaxing agent, Asian ginseng has an invigorating effect, making Korean Red Ginseng a preferred choice for those who need an energy boost.

Living in the backwoods of Nova Scotia, it's not easy to find Korean Red Ginseng in my local area, but I have found a reliable source that delivers it to my doorstep. I take a quarter tip of a spoon once a week, and during the winter cold and flu season,

It's that simple! If you're looking for a natural and effective way to support your health, I highly recommend giving Korean Red Ginseng a try: goes great with Aswaganda.

.

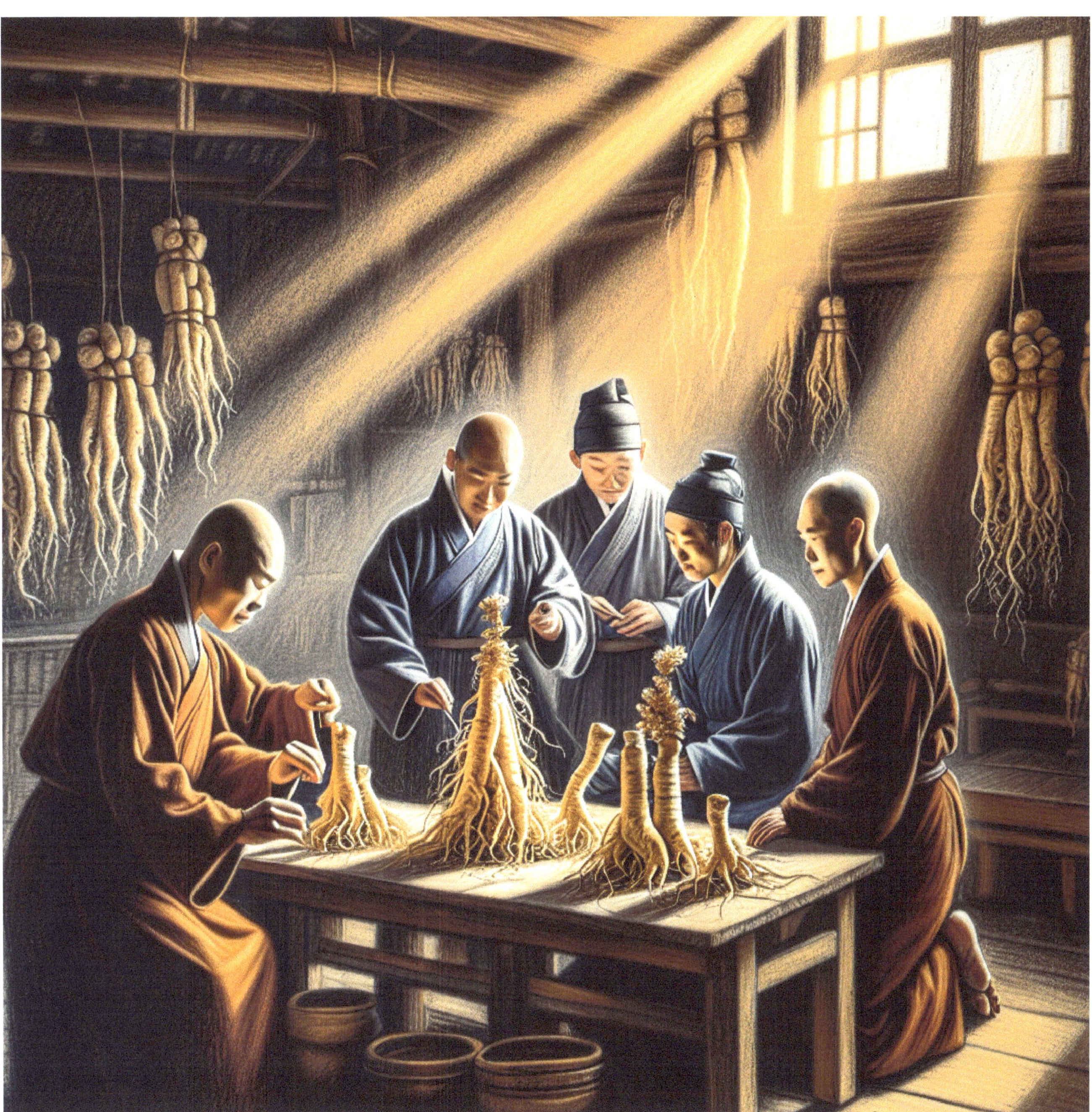

Chapter 3: Cultivating Memory like wow so as to be on top a things all the time with ease

Are you looking for a natural way to enhance your cognitive ability and memory? <u>Lion's Mane mushroom</u> is a powerful and delicious solution. While it can be expensive to buy, growing it at home is an affordable alternative. You only need a wheat straw bale and mycelium spores from Etsy
to get started. Lion's Mane has been recognized in
Chinese culture as a delicious delicacy with a taste similar
to lobster and crab. But it is also known for its cognitive benefits. Regular consumption can help improve your recall and cognitive ability. It's a smart investment to make in yourself. So why not try Lion's Mane today? It's an easy substitute for your daily coffee budget, and the benefits are worth it. Get started on growing your own or buying in bulk from eBay. Lion's Mane is the natural solution you've been looking to find and team up with Cordycep Mushrooms for
an extra cognitive performance edge

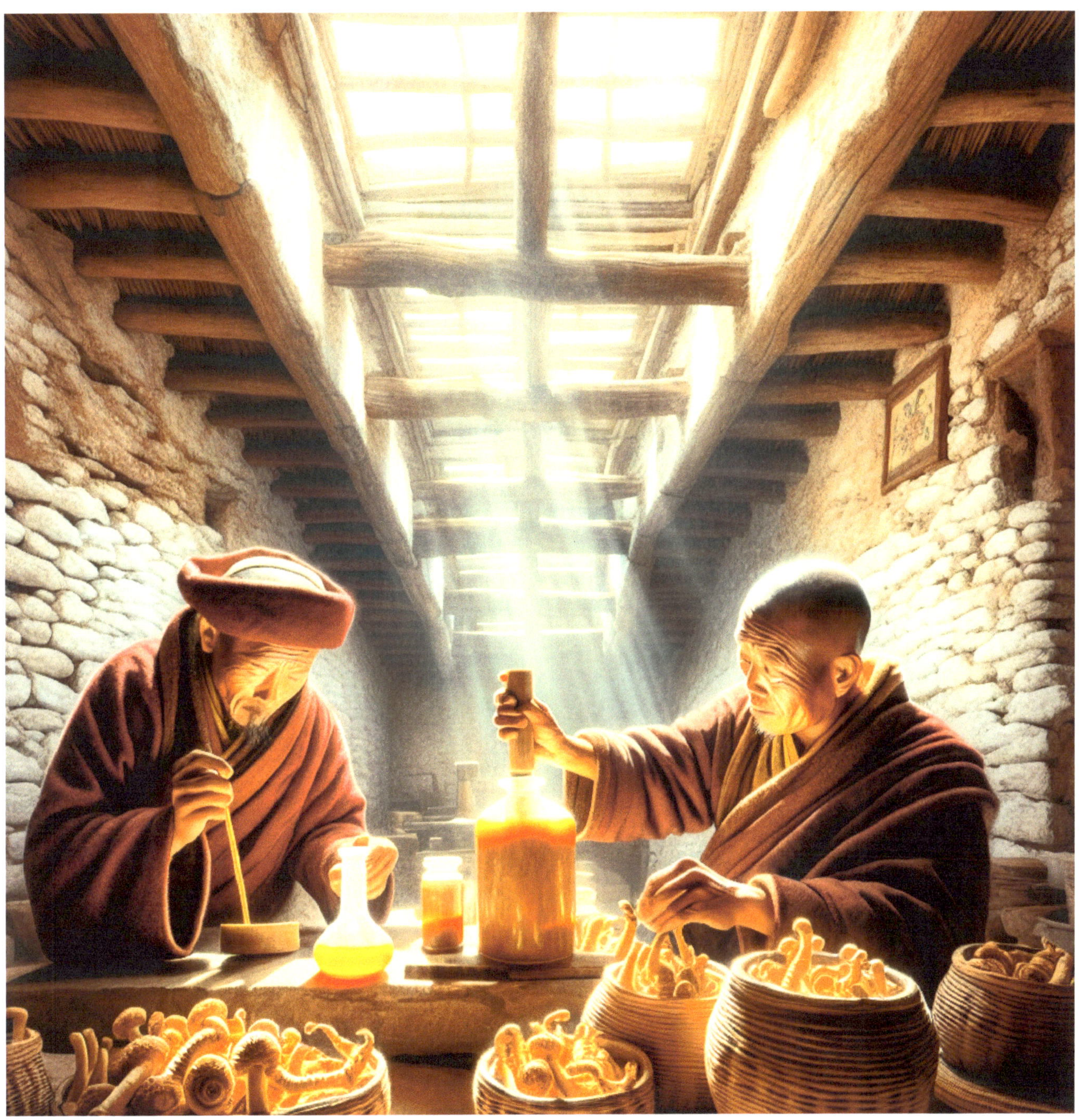

Chapter 4: Royal Jelly for a reason

Royal jelly, often revered as nature's tonic, has captured attention not just for its potential in extending lifespan, but also for its profound support of cognitive well-being. Abundant in vital nutrients, amino acids, and fatty acids, this secretion from honeybee glands presents promising advantages for overall health.

Recent research has shed light on its capacity to foster the growth of neural stem cells, a critical process in brain rejuvenation and upkeep. TCM use royal jelly as a linchpin in staving off cognitive decline by fostering the proliferation of neural stem cells. This groundbreaking revelation holds promise in the battle against age-related cognitive ailments like Alzheimer's disease.

Furthermore, the diverse array of vitamins and antioxidants present in royal jelly could fortify cognitive function by shielding against oxidative stress and inflammation. As we probe deeper into the intricate nexus between nutrition and cognitive well-being, royal jelly emerges as a natural ally in the pursuit of longevity and mental sharpness.

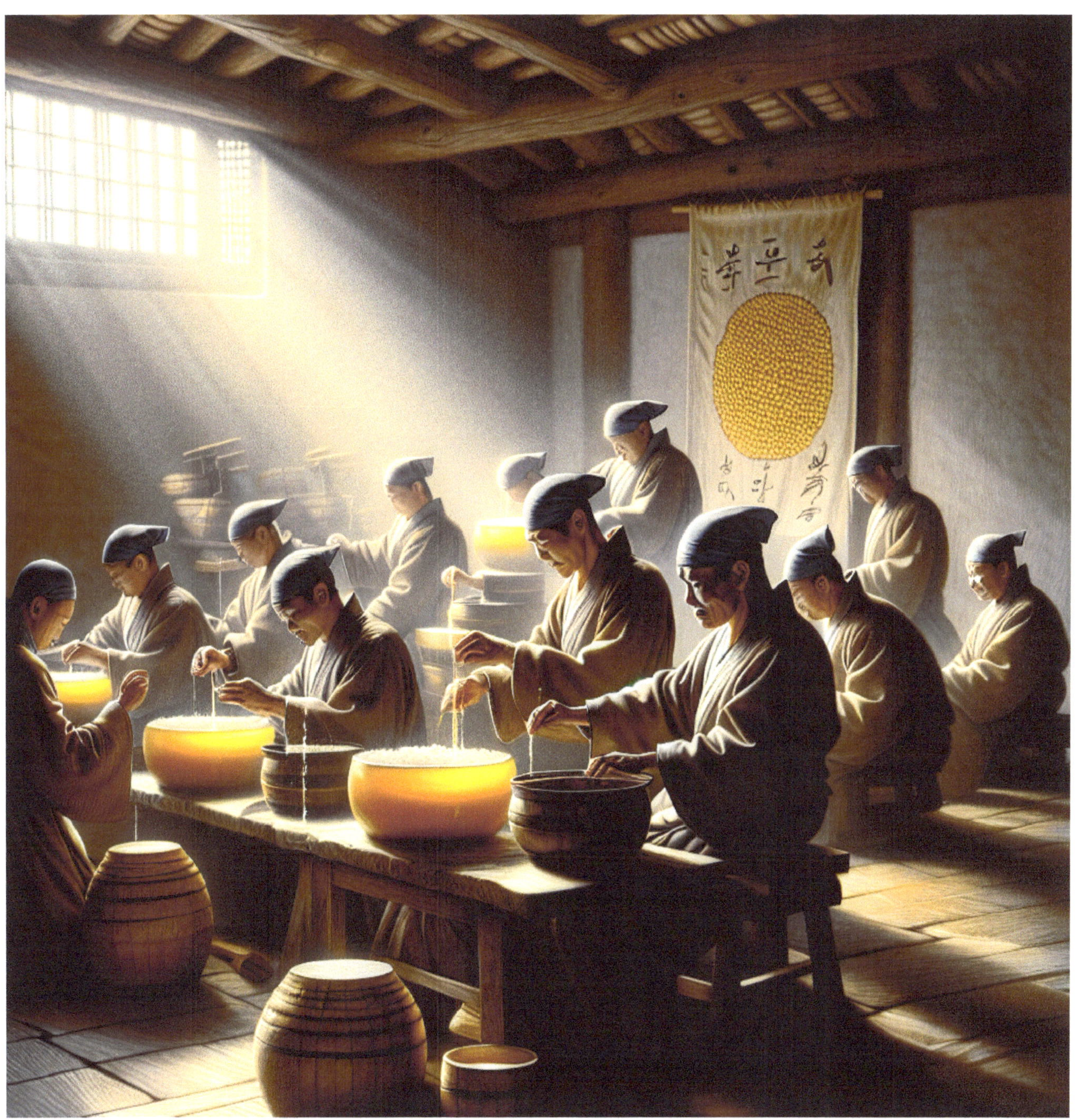

Chapter 5: Morning Wood Solution:
Reviving the spirited stallion named Mornin`wood
and returning him to the stable of Daddi.

Deer antler velvet stands as a revered remedy in traditional Chinese medicine, renowned for its multitude of health benefits. Among its most notable attributes is its rich concentration of growth factors. These natural proteins, inherent to our bodies, play a pivotal role in fostering cell growth, repair, and rejuvenation. By incorporating deer antler velvet into Mornin`wood's wellness regimen, we can tap into the potency of these growth factors to bolster his overall health and vigor.

Furthermore, deer antler velvet serves as a veritable reservoir of essential nutrients. It boasts an extensive array of amino acids, the fundamental components IGF-1 night crew;crucial for diverse bodily functions. Additionally, it brims with glycosaminoglycans, vital for maintaining joint health and cartilage integrity. Moreover, this natural solution is brimming with minerals and trace elements, offering comprehensive support for optimal well-being.

Integrating deer antler velvet into your daily routine can provide a holistic approach to nurturing his wellness, fortifying cellular function, and enhancing his overall vitality.

Available in supplement form or sliced for convenient incorporation into morning tisanes.

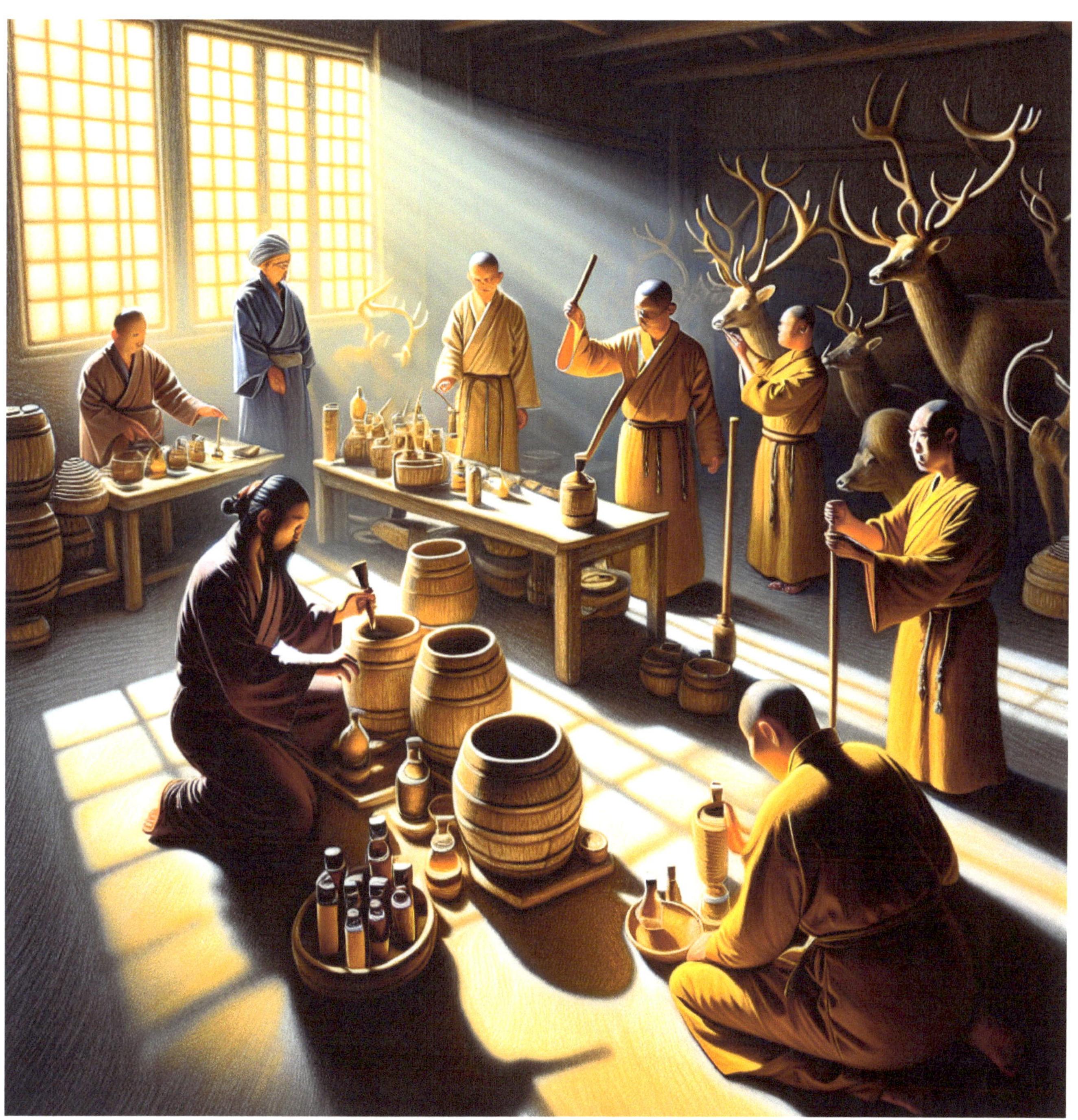

Chapter 6: Dynamics of Stem cells

The potential of stem cell technology continues to captivate researchers and enthusiasts alike. From regenerating tissues to revitalizing organs, the possibilities seem boundless. A notable figure in this field is Ben Greenfield, whose full spinal documentary sheds light on the transformative power of stem cells, particularly in regenerating the dorsal spinal column, akin to the backbone of the Tree of Life.
Greenfield's work illuminates how this regeneration extends beyond mere structural repair, permeating through the torso trunk organs, revitalizing and rejuvenating the body. It's a remarkable testament to the regenerative capacity inherent in stem cells, offering hope for those grappling with degenerative conditions and injuries.
The implications are profound for individuals seeking to optimize their health and well-being. Stem cell potential is something to aim for, a beacon of hope on the horizon of medical progress.
Moreover, the integration of stem cell technology into skincare highlights its versatility and applicability. High-quality stem cell technology is making its way into skincare products, promising rejuvenation and regeneration at the cellular level. It's a testament to the expanding horizons of stem cell research, reaching beyond traditional medical applications into the realm of cosmetic enhancement.offering new avenues for enhancing health and vitality now.

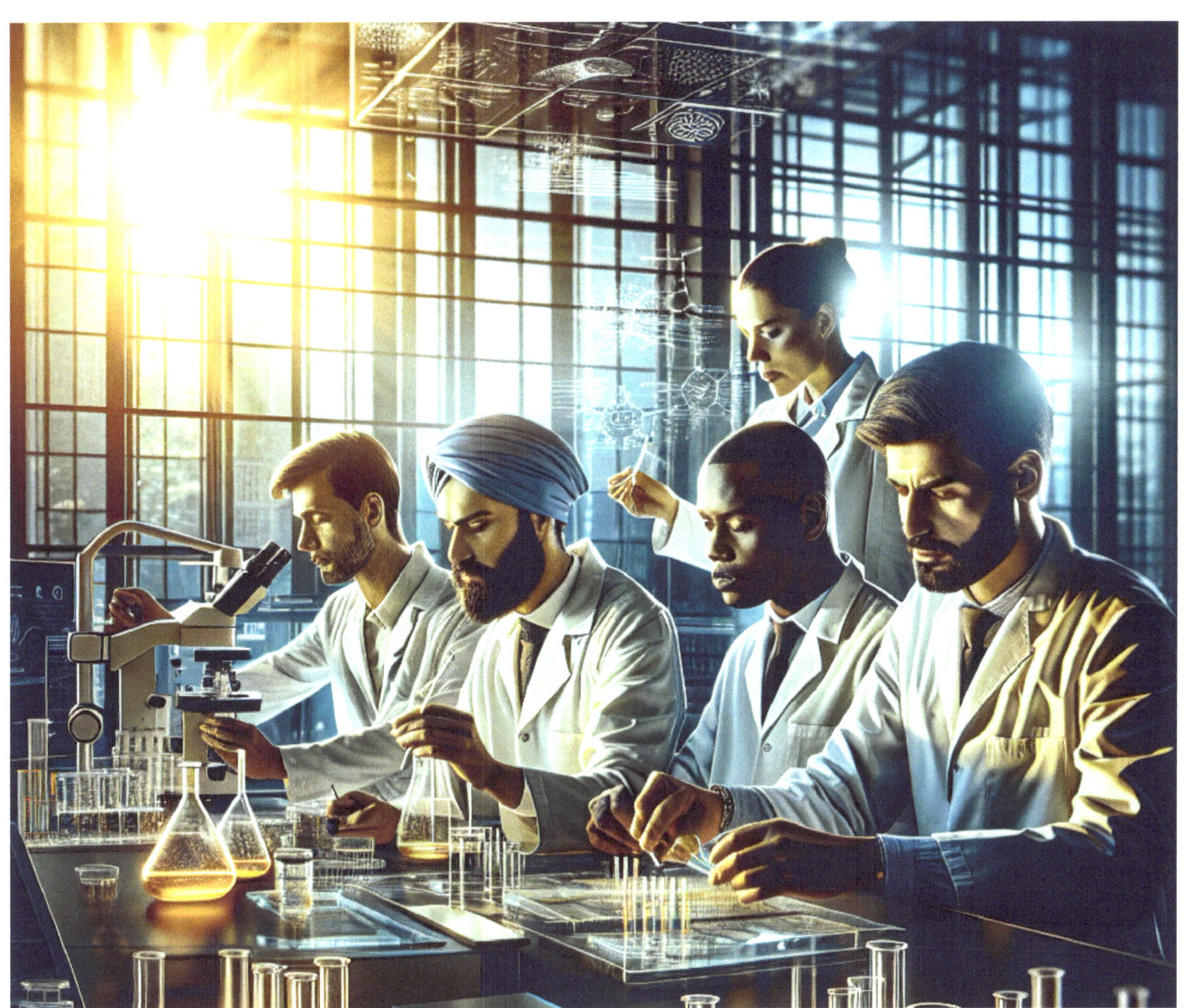

Chapter 7: Unlocking the Secrets of Argan Oil: A Moroccan Treasure for Hair and Health

Argan oil has long been hailed as a beauty elixir, revered for its myriad of benefits for both hair and skin. Originating from Morocco, this organic oil undergoes a meticulous extraction process, ensuring purity and potency. The first press yields the most concentrated and nutrient-rich oil, retaining its essence.. Argan oil isn't just a beauty staple; its versatility extends to culinary uses too. Make it becomes a valuable cost effective addition to your regimen. Rich in essential fatty acids, antioxidants, and vitamins, it nourishes and hydrates the scalp and hair, promoting strength and shine.

Moreover, the culinary potential of Argan oil is equally remarkable. Blend it with vinegar and herbs to create a revitalizing salad dressing. This infusion not only tantalizes the taste buds but also supports inner well-being, thanks to the oil's nutritional profile.

Whether you're seeking to rejuvenate your hair or enhance your culinary creations, Argan oil stands as a testament to the natural wonders found in the heart of Morocco. Embrace this ancient treasure and experience its transformative power firsthand.

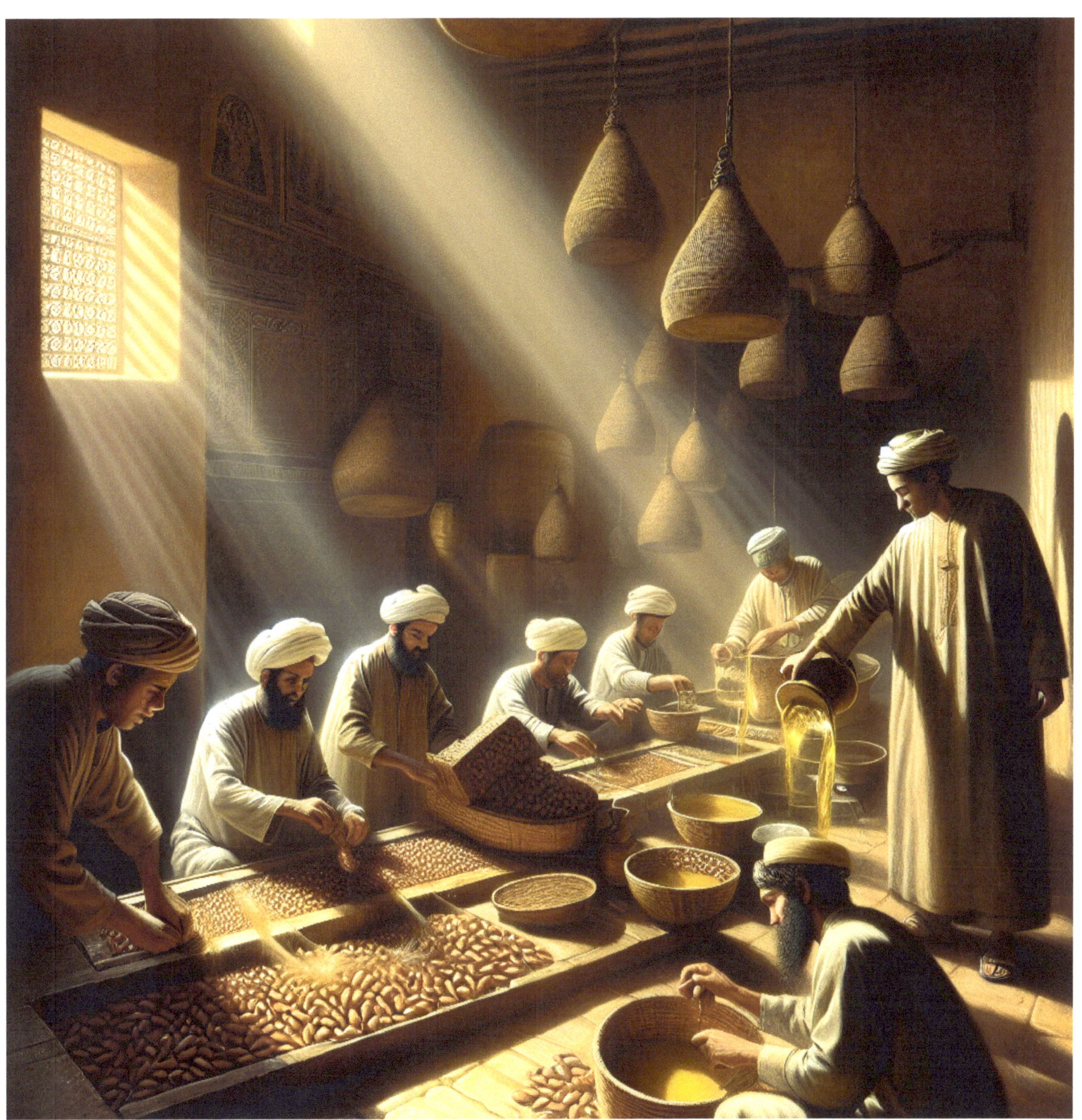

**Chapter 8: Body scrub away
the emotional static cling**

In just five minutes, experience an unparalleled pick-me-up with a good body Scrub to reboot yourself. Simply wet, turn off shower ,smeer all over,wipe, and rinse, and feel the rejuvenating effects on your skin. Look for s good blend of sugar, sea salt, and coffee grounds; since that is the combo that offers a refreshing exfoliation that leaves your skin feeling polished and revitalized.

I am not keen on a <u>big Honkin`Man Scrub Jar</u> , perfect for those seeking a budget-friendly option. Elevate your scrubbing experience by adding a layer of shea butter after the coffee scrub; since your skin is still warm and capable of absorbing the shea butter.
Indulge in this luxurious skincare ritual and discover the transformative experience the Spa industry charges lots for. Since it literally removes the emotional static cling of of ya`.

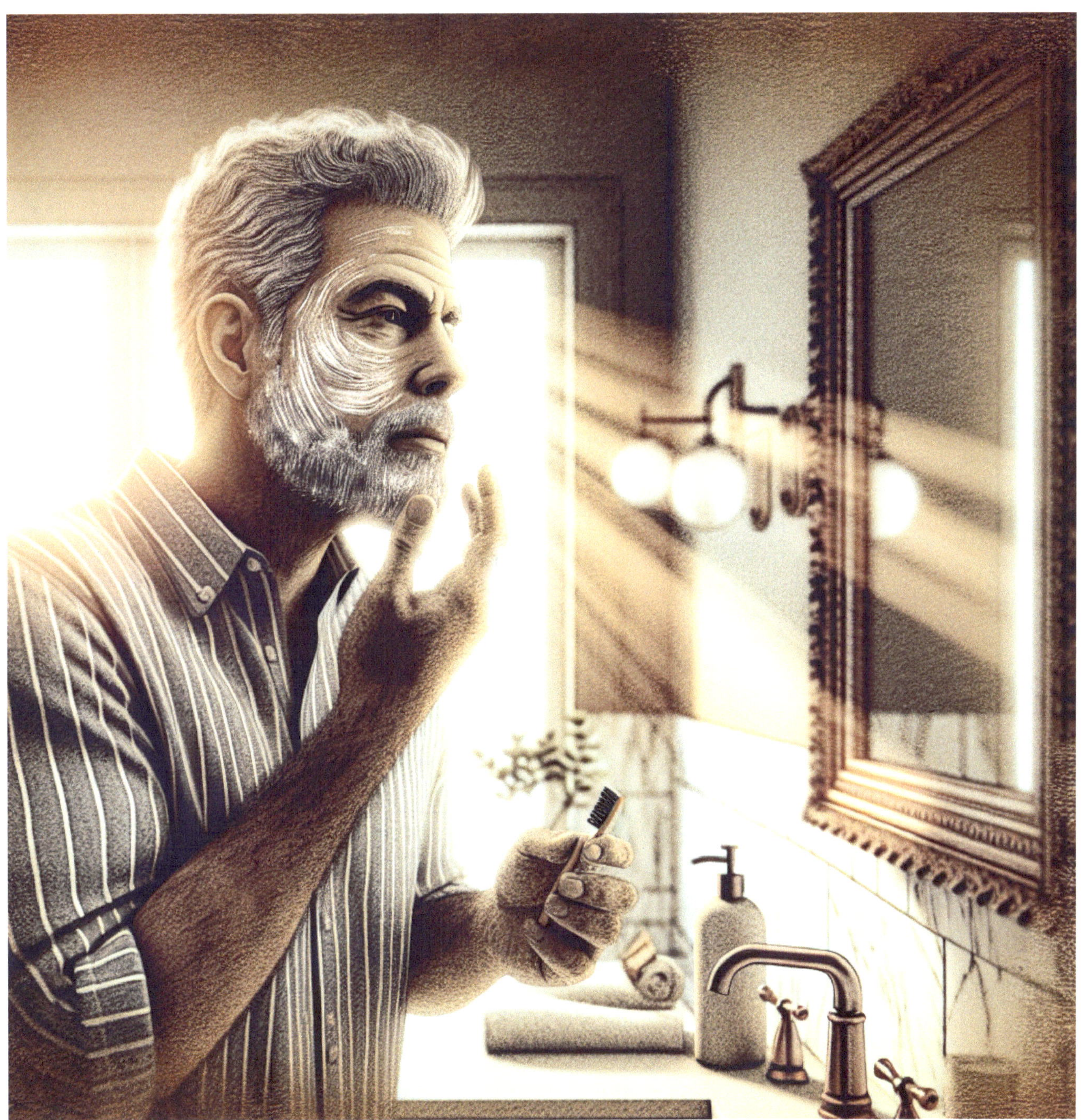

Chapter 9: Guts of steel

Nourish Your Gut for Optimal Well-Being

A flourishing stomach is the cornerstone of overall health, especially for those who relish their meals. With unwavering confidence, I boast what some may call "guts of steel." The
cycle of eating, digestion, and elimination harmoniously unfolds, thanks to the insights of Dr. Steven Gundry. His expertise surpasses my own, prompting me to secure an account with his platform.

This affiliation grants exclusive access to invaluable resources, including a 50% discount on launch deals and priority access to groundbreaking advancements in bioaccessible nutrition for the gastrointestinal tract. It's the ultimate hub for sourcing top-tier supplements, with frequent flash sales offering discounts ranging from 30% to 58%.

Dr. Gundry's teachings illuminate the intricate workings of gut health, underscoring its pivotal role in overall well-being. By prioritizing the nourishment of our digestive system, we lay the foundation for a vibrant and resilient body. Join me in embracing this journey towards optimal GI tract health, sourced from the expertise of Dr. Gundry's platform.

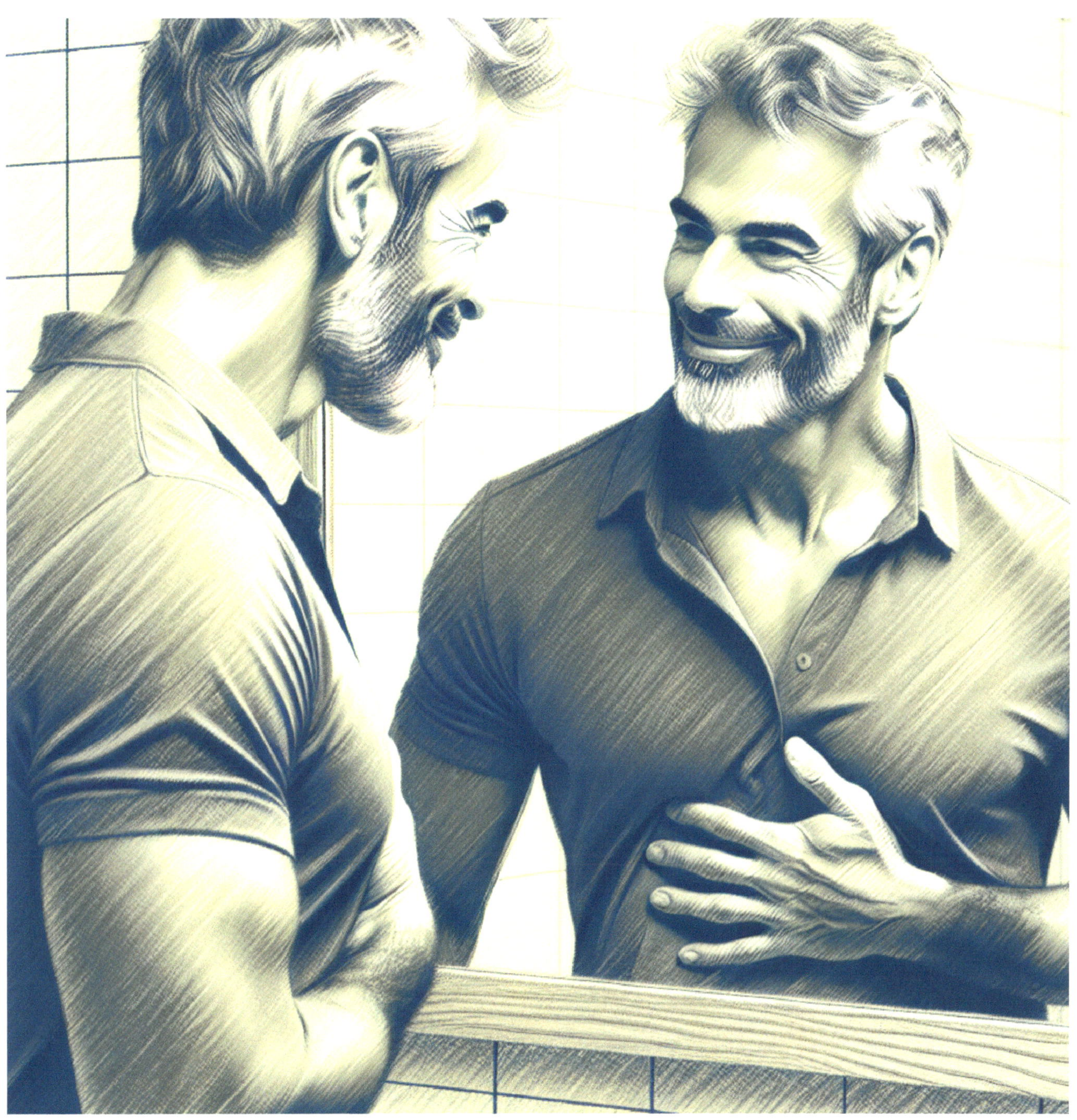

Chapter 10: Far Infrared and you

Time Tested Power of Nikken Far Infrared Magnet Technology

Nikken's far infrared magnet technology has been a game-changer for over five decades, generating immense value, reaching into the trillions of dollars. The reason behind this success lies in the exceptional quality of their magnet insoles, a product that has become synonymous with comfort and support. Fortunately, online offers a convenient platform to access these products through Nikken's worldwide distributor network.

Beyond their renowned magnet insoles, Nikken offers a range of exceptional products designed to enhance nutrition and sleep quality. From personal experience, I can attest to the effectiveness of their sleep system, which I've enjoyed on my massage table for years. While these products boast superior quality, they do come with a higher price tag and are exclusively available through Nikken's network of distributors.

Although Nikken operates through a multi-level marketing (MLM) model, making it inaccessible through traditional retail outlets, the online marketplace provides a cost-effective avenue to access their innovative Kenko technology. With its unparalleled energy benefits, Nikken's products are certainly worth exploring for those seeking enhanced well-being. Dive
into the research and discover the transformative potential
of Nikken's energy technology.

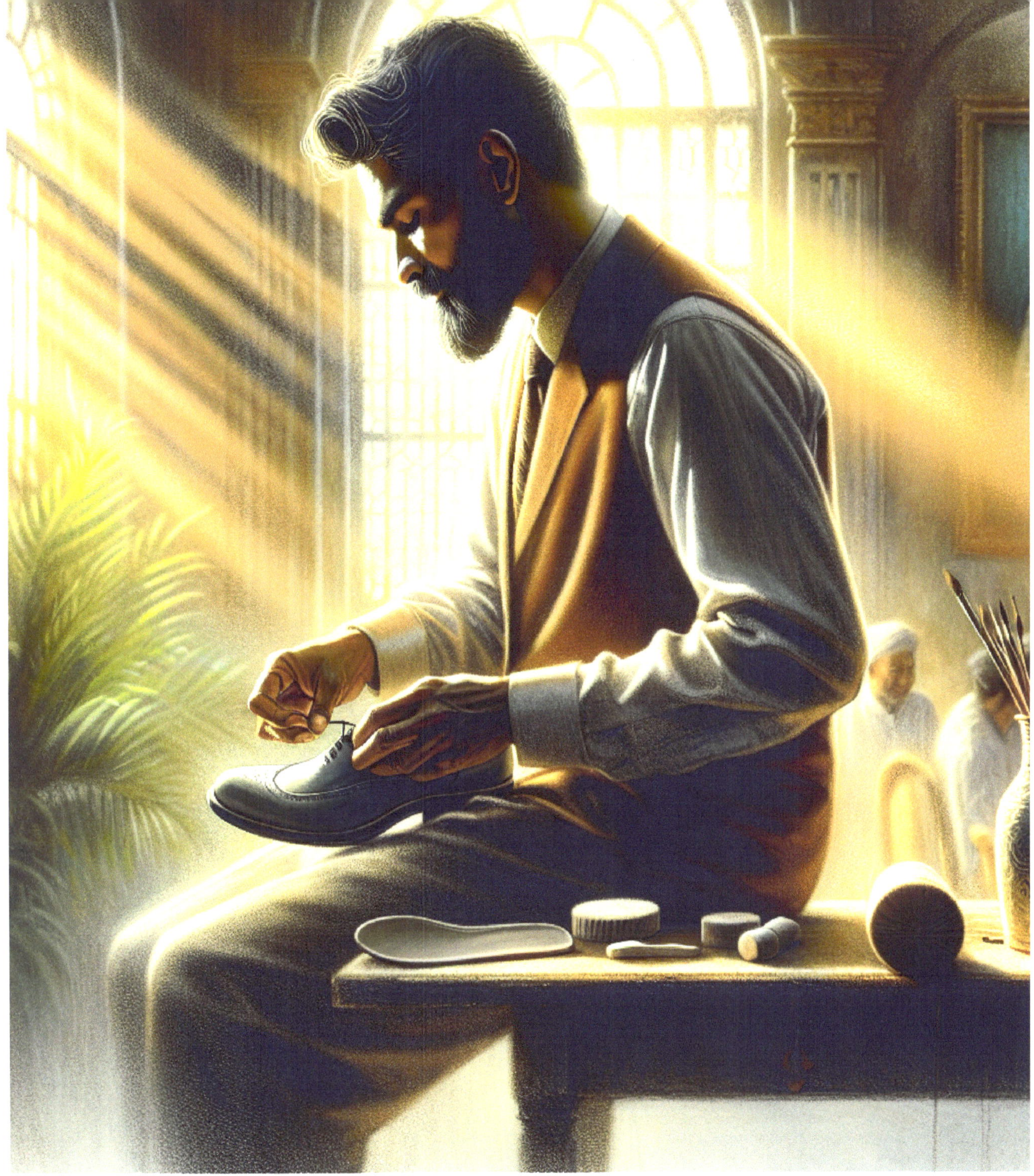

Chapter 11: Tourmaline gemstone heat mats: .

You need to hit the ground running every morning. Tourmaline, a semi-precious mineral renowned for its therapeutic properties, has gained popularity for its ability to emit far infrared rays and negative ions. These natural elements are known to stimulate the body's healing process, leading to improved blood circulation and relief from pain and inflammation.

<u>Tourmaline heating pads, which emit far infrared</u>, have been found to boost the immune system and aid in detoxification. This electromagnetic radiation promotes cellular metabolism and increases alertness, contributing to overall well-being. Additionally, tourmaline possesses grounding properties that induce relaxation and enhance emotional stability.

The benefits of are extensive, ranging from weight loss and reduced water retention to improved liver and kidney function. They are particularly beneficial for alleviating back and neck pain, muscle stiffness, joint pain, and spasms

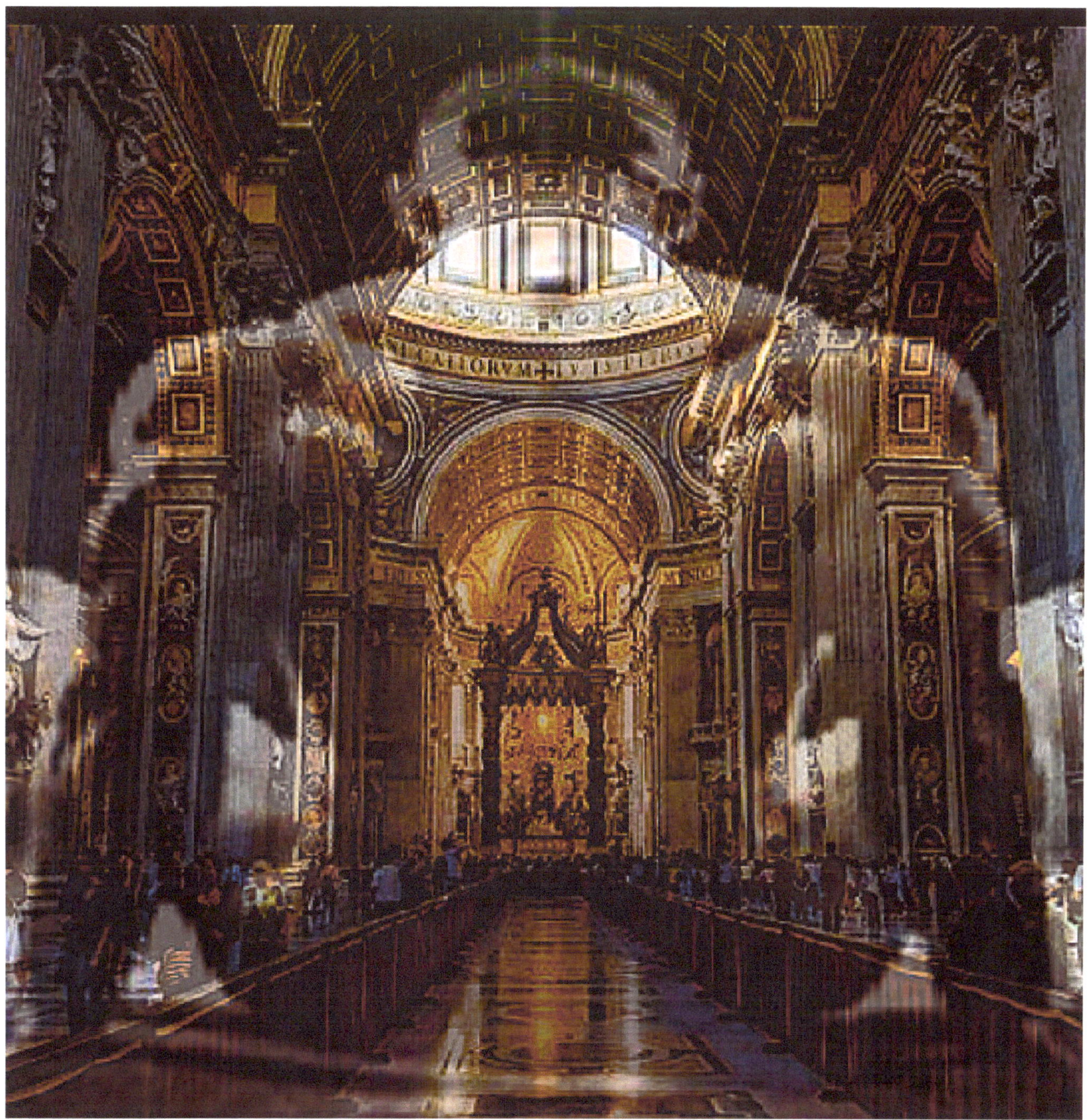

Chapter 12: Haelo PEMF device.

The <u>Haelo PEMF device</u> isn't just a gadget; it's a game-changer in the realms of recovery and performance enhancement. Its innovative approach underscores the inseparable link between the two, emphasizing that optimal performance is attainable with proper recovery strategies.

Sporting a sleek circular design with a generous 6-foot radius for multiple individuals to experience its rejuvenating effects simultaneously. It boasts an impressive array of 14 different settings, including options for regeneration and invigoration, and users can seamlessly alternate between modes for a comprehensive wellness experience.

While this cutting-edge device may come with a price tag, it's undoubtedly an investment in one's well-being. So, if you're eyeing it for your holiday wish list, it might be time to consider a side hustle to boost your finances. After all, the benefits it promises are worth every penny.

So, this Christmas, why not treat yourself or a loved one to the gift of enhanced recovery and performance with the Haelo PEMF device? It's a present that promises long-lasting health and vitality, making it a worthy addition to any holiday shopping list.

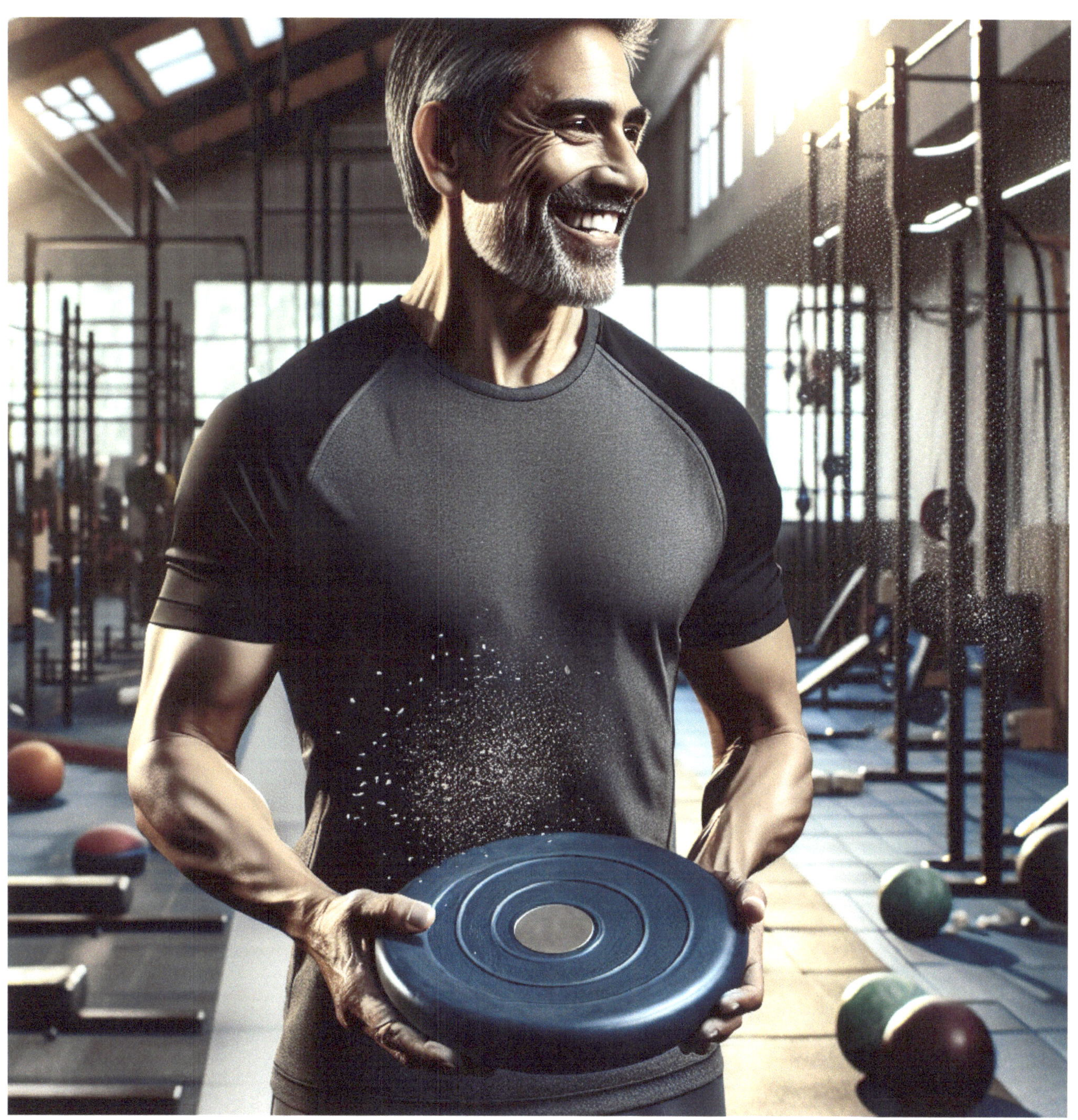

Chapter 13: The Spooky 2 Scalar device

It has caught my attention, aligning perfectly with my interest in integrating technology, nutrition, and mindfulness practices. It offers a unique approach to calming the mind and enhancing focus, essential for achieving goals with clarity.

As I eagerly await their upcoming 20% Black Friday sale in November, I'm excited about the prospect of saving $400 off its $2,100 price tag. Once I acquire it, I'll be sure to provide an update on my experience.
The Spooky 2 Scalar operates by transmitting a back-and-forth signal. This process effectively creates a scalar field, fostering an environment conducive to regeneration for the body's 37 trillion mitochondria. What's remarkable is that this rejuvenating session takes just 25-45 minutes and can accommodate multiple individuals between the transmitter and receiver.
While some may label it as "woo-woo," the benefits are undeniable. Start using the Spooky 2 Scalar and witnessing firsthand its positive impact on overall well-being.

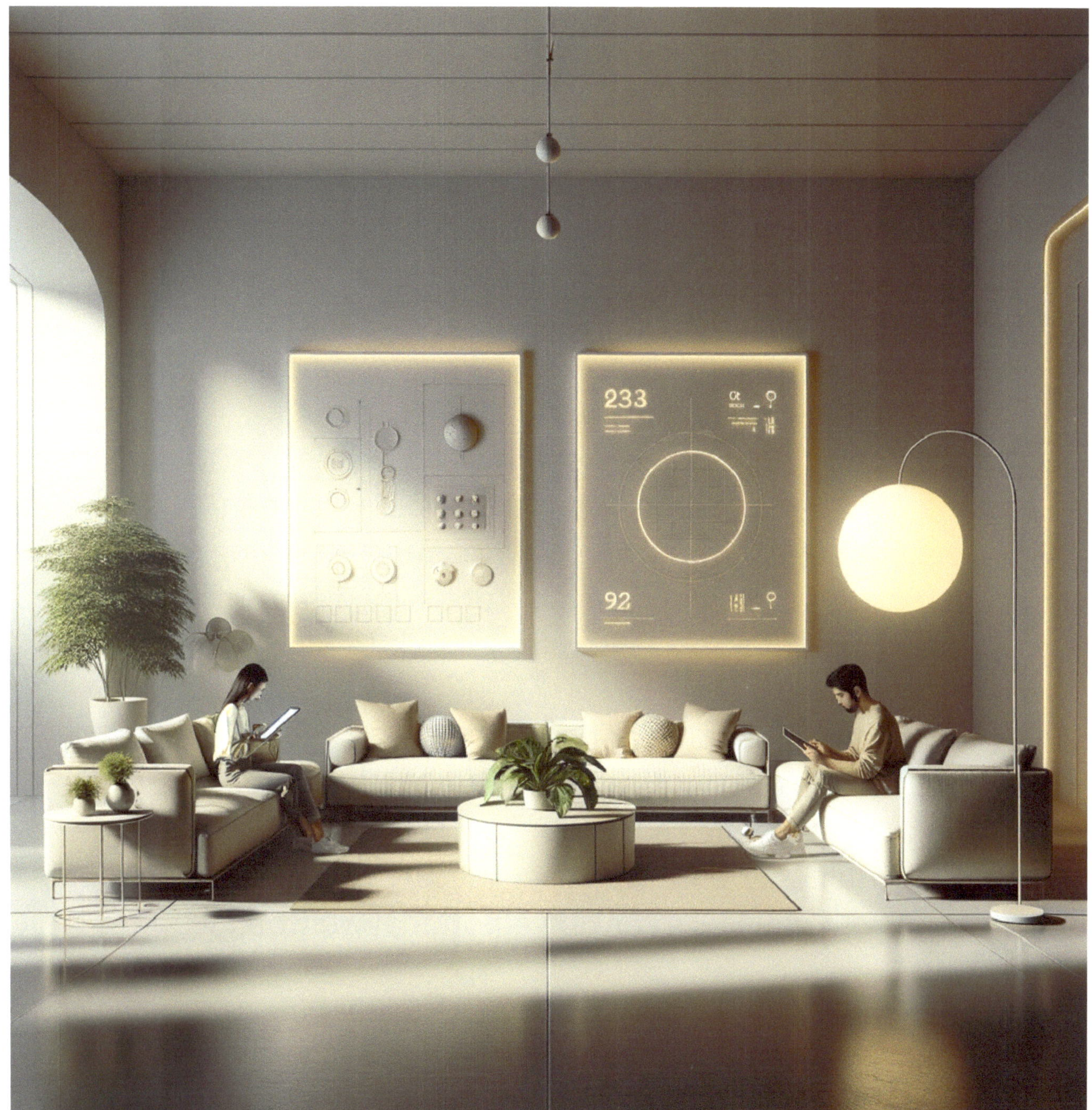

233
92

Chapter 14: Two minute Tapping solution

The Tapping Solution, also known as Emotional Freedom Technique (EFT), emerges as an indispensable mind-body tool offering remarkable benefits at no cost. Just two minutes here and there can work wonders for alleviating anxiety, aiding smoking cessation, managing PTSD, and addressing a myriad of other issues.

Nick Ortner, alongside his sister Jessica Ortner, provides an abundance of free resources on their YouTube channel. These video walkthroughs offer practical guidance, reaching millions of individuals worldwide. The content they offer is not only accessible but also easy to integrate into daily routines.

EFT involves simply tapping on specific points on the face, hands, collarbone, and head. Despite its simplicity, this technique delivers profound therapeutic relief from various forms of distress. Its essential nature and cost-free accessibility make it an invaluable tool for anyone seeking emotional well-being.

With the ability to reuse and reapply as needed, the Tapping Solution app stands as a beacon of hope, offering effective relief from life's challenges through a straightforward and accessible approach.

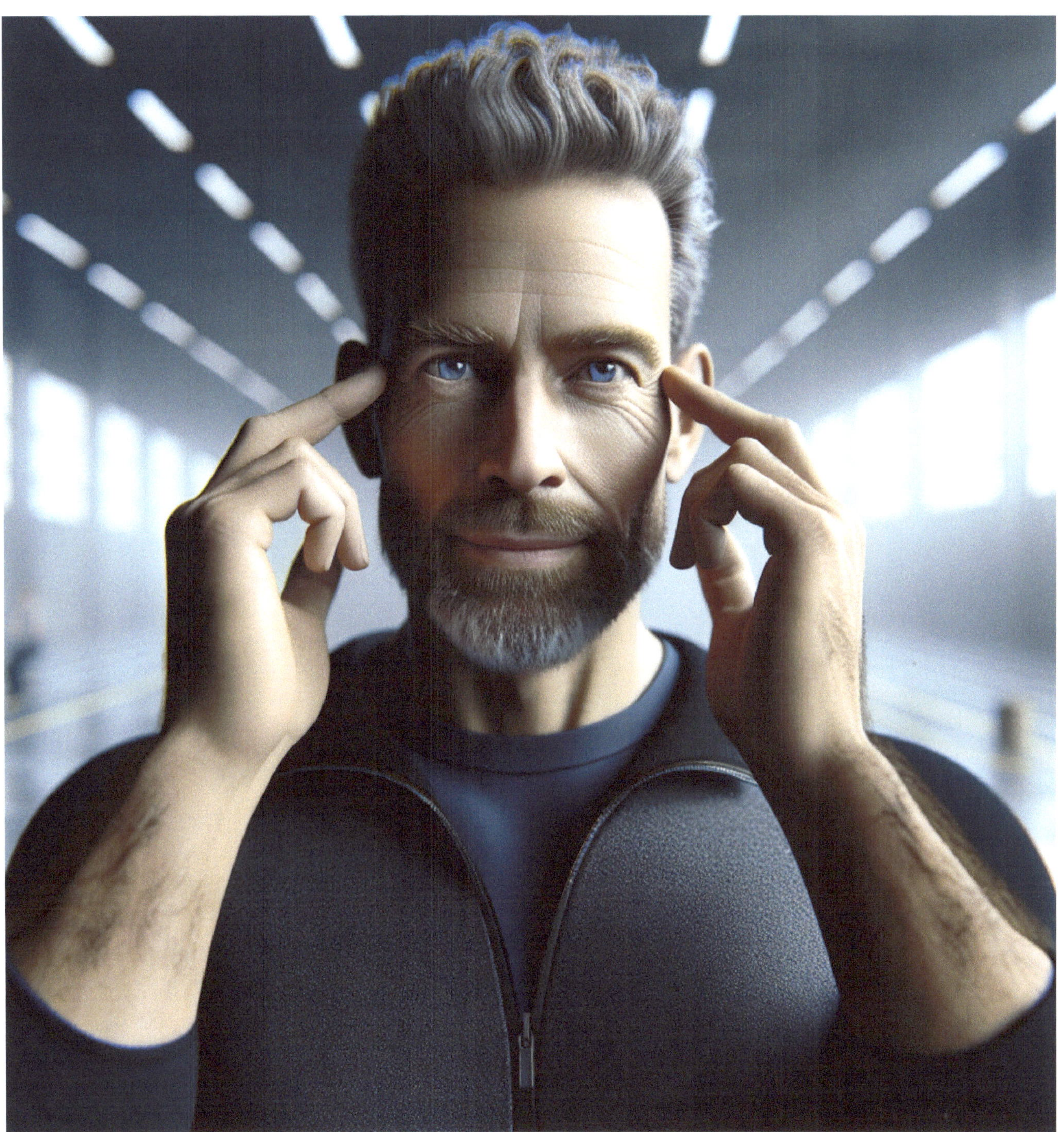

Chapter 15: Breathwork, guided by experts like hypnotherapist Marisa Peer or with the soothing voice of Paul McKenna

Breathwork facilitates deep states of release and transformation through techniques that engage every nerve and synchronize both hemispheres of the brain.

Platforms like the Mindvalley app provide access to these high-quality sessions for free, making serious therapeutic experiences accessible to all.
For those seeking a quantum shift, Dr. Jean Houston's breathwork methods offer a pathway to profound change, allowing individuals to release burdens and reclaim their essence.
While some may view these modalities as unconventional, their efficacy is backed by centuries of practice by various cultures worldwide. The wisdom of ancient traditions underscores the profound impact breathwork can have on human optimization and well-being.

Once you've experienced the transformative power of breathwork, mundane distractions like mainstream news lose their grip. Continuously exploring these practices is essential, and I invite you to join me on this journey of growth and discovery.

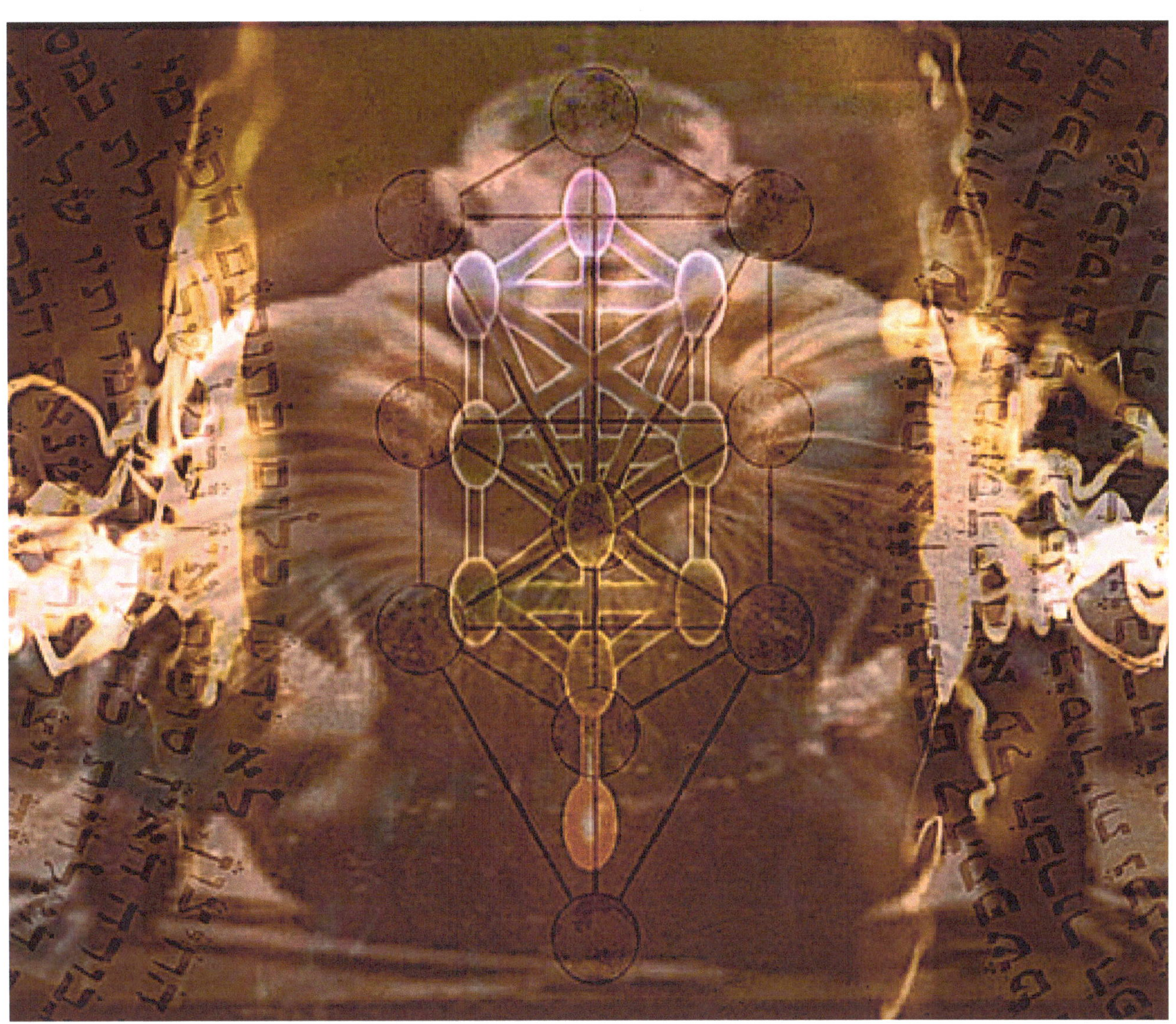

Chapter 16: Once you move forward
you never look back

To get the body stamina and strength youn need theese days , go get a <u>Visionbody Powersuit</u>: a revolutionary advancement in wearable EMS technology. Unlike its predecessors, this cutting-edge suit boasts a completely wireless design, ensuring unparalleled convenience for users. Crafted as a second skin, its innovative design features 20 soft silicone pulse areas strategically placed to target muscles throughout the body. These areas administer a blend of low, middle, and high-frequency EMS pulses, effectively stimulating muscles at their deepest levels.
What sets the Visionbody Powersuit apart is its ability to replicate the muscle contractions experienced during rigorous workouts without imposing strain on joints, tendons, or ligaments. This means you can achieve the benefits of an intense workout with minimal risk of injury.

With over a decade of experience pioneering EMS technology, Visionbody has continually pushed the boundaries of innovation. Whether you're an athlete looking to enhance performance, a fitness enthusiast seeking efficient muscle activation, or someone simply interested in optimizing their workouts, the Visionbody Powersuit offers a game-changing solution. Theyn have financing available and you can channel your solopreneur spirit and sell the serivce

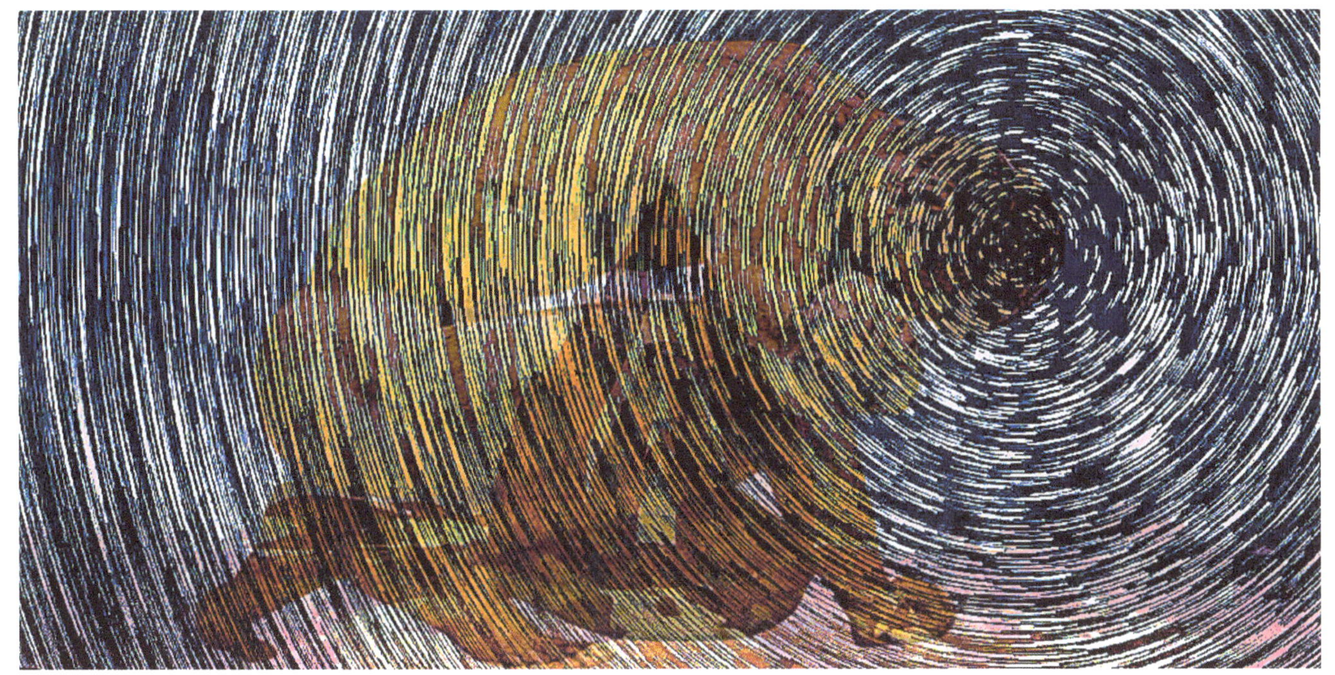

With mindfulness to get rid of the clatter and clutter and focus in on living your best life with the 15 essentails you need to get you to the church on time.
Just like this '4x4 Method' or 'Box Breathing'.
First, exhale completely, pushing out every bit of air.
Inhale quietly through the nose for a calm count of four.
Hold that breath gently, letting the silence fill you for another four counts.Exhale slowly, allowing a count of four to guide the release.Pause at the bottom of your exhale, counting to four once more.
Perform this sequence four times, or continue until you feel the calm settle in.

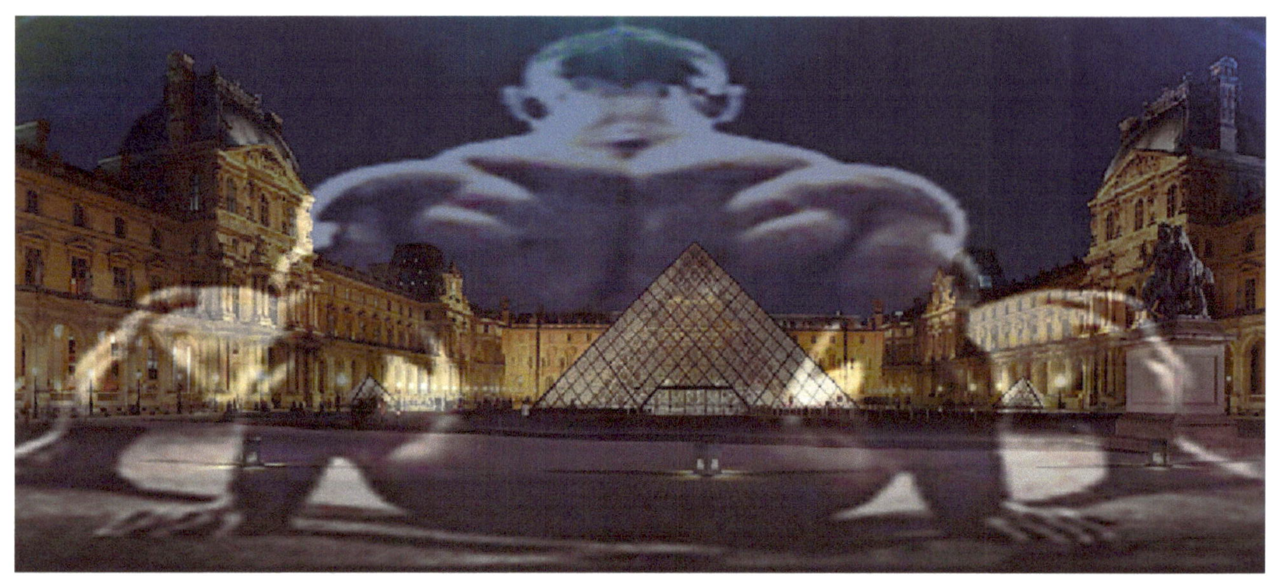

As you synchronize your breath with the rhythmic motion of the compass bow rotational cycle depicted in these exquisite motion graphics, distractions fade away, allowing you to enter a state of flow.

This immersive practice liberates you from the clutter of thoughts and distractions, enabling you to tap into your inner potential and pursue your life's purpose with clarity and focus. By aligning your breath with the visual cues provided by the Mandala Mudra and Theriault's motion graphics, you embark on a journey of self-discovery and optimization.

www.ingramcontent.com/pod-product-compliance
Lightning Source LLC
Chambersburg PA
CBHW040201240726
48664CB00002B/791